17 DAY DIET

Blank Cook Book

FAST TRACK

WEIGHT LOSS

Speedy Publishing LLC
40 E. Main St., #1156
Newark, DE 19711

www.SpeedyPublishing.Co

Copyright 2014
978-1-63287-912-7
First Printed April 18, 2014

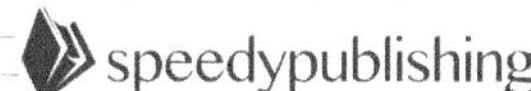

Recipe Name: ____

Ingredient List

....

....

....

....

....

....

....

Cooking Instructions

....

....

....

....

....

....

....

....

About This Dish

Calories: **Fat:**

Protein: **Carbs:**

Personal Rating: ○ ○ ○ ○ ○

Ingredient List

Cooking Instructions

About This Dish

Calories:

Fat:

Protein:

Carbs:

Personal Rating: ○ ○ ○ ○ ○

Recipe Name:

Ingredient List

....

....

....

....

....

....

....

Cooking Instructions

....

....

....

....

....

....

....

About This Dish

Calories: **Fat:**

Protein: **Carbs:**

Personal Rating: ○ ○ ○ ○ ○

Recipe Name: ____

Ingredient List

....

....

....

....

....

....

....

Cooking Instructions

....

....

....

....

....

....

....

....

About This Dish

Calories: **Fat:**

Protein: **Carbs:**

Personal Rating: ○ ○ ○ ○ ○

Recipe Name:

Ingredient List

Cooking Instructions

About This Dish

Calories:

Fat:

Protein:

Carbs:

Personal Rating: ○ ○ ○ ○ ○

Recipe Name:

Ingredient List

Cooking Instructions

About This Dish

Calories:

Fat:

Protein:

Carbs:

Personal Rating: ○ ○ ○ ○ ○

Recipe Name: ....

Ingredient List

....

....

....

....

....

....

....

....

Cooking Instructions

....

....

....

....

....

....

....

....

About This Dish

Calories: **Fat:**

Protein: **Carbs:**

Personal Rating: ○ ○ ○ ○ ○

Recipe Name:

Ingredient List

Cooking Instructions

About This Dish

Calories:

Fat:

Protein:

Carbs:

Personal Rating: ○ ○ ○ ○ ○

Recipe Name: ....

Ingredient List

....
....
....
....
....
....
....

Cooking Instructions

....
....
....
....
....
....
....
....

About This Dish

Calories: **Fat:**

Protein: **Carbs:**

Personal Rating: ○ ○ ○ ○ ○

Recipe Name:

Ingredient List

Cooking Instructions

About This Dish

Calories:

Fat:

Protein:

Carbs:

Personal Rating: ○ ○ ○ ○ ○

Recipe Name:

Ingredient List

Cooking Instructions

About This Dish

Calories:

Fat:

Protein:

Carbs:

Personal Rating: ○ ○ ○ ○ ○

Recipe Name:

Ingredient List

Cooking Instructions

About This Dish

Calories:

Fat:

Protein:

Carbs:

Personal Rating: ○ ○ ○ ○ ○

Recipe Name: ....

Ingredient List

....
....
....
....
....
....
....

Cooking Instructions

....
....
....
....
....
....
....
....

About This Dish

Calories: **Fat:**

Protein: **Carbs:**

Personal Rating: ○ ○ ○ ○ ○

Ingredient List

Cooking Instructions

About This Dish

Calories:

Fat:

Protein:

Carbs:

Personal Rating: ○ ○ ○ ○ ○

Recipe Name: ....

Ingredient List

....

....

....

....

....

....

....

....

Cooking Instructions

....

....

....

....

....

....

....

....

About This Dish

Calories: **Fat:**

Protein: **Carbs:**

Personal Rating: ◯ ◯ ◯ ◯ ◯

Recipe Name:

Ingredient List

Cooking Instructions

About This Dish

Calories:

Fat:

Protein:

Carbs:

Personal Rating: ○ ○ ○ ○ ○

Recipe Name: ____

Ingredient List

Cooking Instructions

About This Dish

Calories:

Fat:

Protein:

Carbs:

Personal Rating: ○ ○ ○ ○ ○

Recipe Name: ....

Ingredient List

....
....
....
....
....
....
....
....

Cooking Instructions

....
....
....
....
....
....
....
....

About This Dish

Calories:

Fat:

Protein:

Carbs:

Personal Rating: ○ ○ ○ ○ ○

Recipe Name:

Ingredient List

Cooking Instructions

About This Dish

Calories:

Fat:

Protein:

Carbs:

Personal Rating: ○ ○ ○ ○ ○

Recipe Name:

Ingredient List

Cooking Instructions

About This Dish

Calories: **Fat:**

Protein: **Carbs:**

Personal Rating: ◯ ◯ ◯ ◯ ◯

Recipe Name:

Ingredient List

Cooking Instructions

About This Dish

Calories:

Fat:

Protein:

Carbs:

Personal Rating: ○ ○ ○ ○ ○

Recipe Name:

Ingredient List

Cooking Instructions

About This Dish

Calories:

Fat:

Protein:

Carbs:

Personal Rating: ○ ○ ○ ○ ○

Recipe Name:

Ingredient List

Cooking Instructions

About This Dish

Calories:

Fat:

Protein:

Carbs:

Personal Rating: ○ ○ ○ ○ ○

Recipe Name:

Ingredient List

Cooking Instructions

About This Dish

Calories:

Fat:

Protein:

Carbs:

Personal Rating: ◯ ◯ ◯ ◯ ◯

Recipe Name:

Ingredient List

Cooking Instructions

About This Dish

Calories:

Fat:

Protein:

Carbs:

Personal Rating: ◯ ◯ ◯ ◯ ◯

Recipe Name: ____

Ingredient List

....
....
....
....
....
....
....

Cooking Instructions

....
....
....
....
....
....
....
....

About This Dish

Calories:

Fat:

Protein:

Carbs:

Personal Rating: ○ ○ ○ ○ ○

Recipe Name: --

Ingredient List

....

....

....

....

....

....

....

Cooking Instructions

....

....

....

....

....

....

....

About This Dish

Calories: **Fat:**

Protein: **Carbs:**

Personal Rating: ○ ○ ○ ○ ○

Recipe Name: ....

Ingredient List

....

....

....

....

....

....

....

....

Cooking Instructions

....

....

....

....

....

....

....

....

About This Dish

Calories: **Fat:**

Protein: **Carbs:**

Personal Rating: ○ ○ ○ ○ ○

Ingredient List

Cooking Instructions

About This Dish

Calories:

Fat:

Protein:

Carbs:

Personal Rating: ○ ○ ○ ○ ○

Recipe Name: ....

Ingredient List

....

....

....

....

....

....

....

....

Cooking Instructions

....

....

....

....

....

....

....

....

About This Dish

Calories: Fat:

Protein: Carbs:

Personal Rating: ○ ○ ○ ○ ○

Recipe Name: ....

Ingredient List

.... | ....
.... | ....
.... | ....
.... | ....
.... | ....
.... | ....
.... | ....

Cooking Instructions

....
....
....
....
....
....
....
....

About This Dish

Calories:

Fat:

Protein:

Carbs:

Personal Rating: ○ ○ ○ ○ ○

Recipe Name:

Ingredient List

Cooking Instructions

About This Dish

Calories:

Fat:

Protein:

Carbs:

Personal Rating: ○ ○ ○ ○ ○

Recipe Name: ....

Ingredient List

Cooking Instructions

About This Dish

Calories:

Fat:

Protein:

Carbs:

Personal Rating: ○ ○ ○ ○ ○

Recipe Name: ....

Ingredient List

....

....

....

....

....

....

....

Cooking Instructions

....

....

....

....

....

....

....

....

About This Dish

Calories: **Fat:**

Protein: **Carbs:**

Personal Rating: ○ ○ ○ ○ ○

Recipe Name:

Ingredient List

Cooking Instructions

About This Dish

Calories:

Fat:

Protein:

Carbs:

Personal Rating: ○ ○ ○ ○ ○

Recipe Name:

Ingredient List

Cooking Instructions

About This Dish

Calories:

Fat:

Protein:

Carbs:

Personal Rating: ○ ○ ○ ○ ○

Recipe Name:

Ingredient List

Cooking Instructions

About This Dish

Calories:

Fat:

Protein:

Carbs:

Personal Rating: ○ ○ ○ ○ ○

Recipe Name:

Ingredient List

Cooking Instructions

About This Dish

Calories:

Fat:

Protein:

Carbs:

Personal Rating: ○ ○ ○ ○ ○

Recipe Name:

Ingredient List

Cooking Instructions

About This Dish

Calories: Fat:

Protein: Carbs:

Personal Rating: ○ ○ ○ ○ ○

Recipe Name:

Ingredient List

Cooking Instructions

About This Dish

Calories:

Fat:

Protein:

Carbs:

Personal Rating: ○ ○ ○ ○ ○

Recipe Name:

Ingredient List

Cooking Instructions

About This Dish

Calories:

Fat:

Protein:

Carbs:

Personal Rating: ○ ○ ○ ○ ○

Recipe Name: --

Ingredient List

Cooking Instructions

About This Dish

Calories:

Fat:

Protein:

Carbs:

Personal Rating: ◯ ◯ ◯ ◯ ◯

Recipe Name:

Ingredient List

Cooking Instructions

About This Dish

Calories:

Fat:

Protein:

Carbs:

Personal Rating: ○ ○ ○ ○ ○

Recipe Name: ....

Ingredient List

....

....

....

....

....

....

....

Cooking Instructions

....

....

....

....

....

....

....

....

About This Dish

Calories: Fat:

Protein: Carbs:

Personal Rating: ○ ○ ○ ○ ○

Recipe Name:

Ingredient List

Cooking Instructions

About This Dish

Calories:

Fat:

Protein:

Carbs:

Personal Rating: ○ ○ ○ ○ ○

Recipe Name:

Ingredient List

Cooking Instructions

About This Dish

Calories: Fat:

Protein: Carbs:

Personal Rating: ○ ○ ○ ○ ○

Recipe Name:

Ingredient List

Cooking Instructions

About This Dish

Calories:

Fat:

Protein:

Carbs:

Personal Rating: ○ ○ ○ ○ ○

Recipe Name:

Ingredient List

Cooking Instructions

About This Dish

Calories:

Fat:

Protein:

Carbs:

Personal Rating: ○ ○ ○ ○ ○